THE LITTLE BOOK OF
CYCLING

Published by OH!
20 Mortimer Street
London W1T 3JW

ISBN 978-1-80069-006-6

Compiled by: Malcolm Croft
Editorial: Lisa Dyer
Project manager: Russell Porter
Design: Tony Seddon
Production: Freencky Portas

A CIP catalogue record for this book is available from the British Library

Printed in Dubai

10 9 8 7 6 5 4 3 2 1

Illustrations: Freepik.com

THE LITTLE BOOK OF
CYCLING

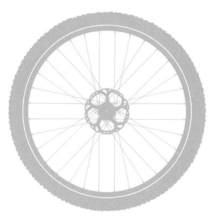

FOR EVERYONE FROM
THE NOVICE TO THE ENTHUSIAST

CONTENTS

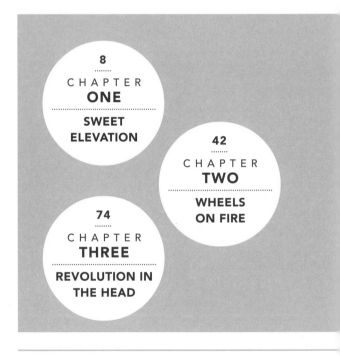

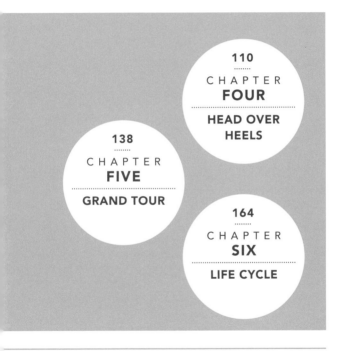

INTRODUCTION

Aero-head. Gear-junkie. Chain-smoker. Chrome pony. Roadie. Wrenchie. Spokie. Lycra lout (or worse, MAMIL – Middle Aged Man in Lycra). Knight Rider. Deliveroo'er. Bikeaholic. Or just plain cyclist. No matter how, or what, you ride, or what you call yourself, if you love the open road and the feeling of wind on both sets of cheeks, then welcome home to *The Little Book of Cycling*. It's the littlest of love letters dedicated to the celebration of all things cycling.

As you'll know, the past two decades have seen the world turn its attention to cycling, in all its two-wheeled forms, more than ever before. Today, getting on your bike is as cool as it is convenient, as awesome as it aspirational, with everyone from presidents to princes and celebrities to commuters going for a spin and taking their trusty Strava or Garmin with them. Even more recent inventions, such as Peloton, SoulCycle and Spin classes – where you can enjoy the medal of the pedal while watching TV – have broken the glass ceiling of cycling, highlighting just how much power the bicycle wields in our modern lives. We are in the midst of a cycling revolution!

Where once getting on your bike was merely a way to go from A to B, being a cyclist is now a way of life, a philosophy ("It's only a hill, get over it!", etc), a proud social status and a term of respect. Your humble carbon-fibre horse has itself become an icon of freedom and possibility, as well as still being a safe, healthy and efficient means of transport.

With all that in mind, *The Little Book of Cycling* is here to take you to school, via bicycle, naturally. It's action-packed with all the facts, stats, quips and quotes that will make your heart and head spin, and it looks great in yellow too. And, pro tip, if you stick the book between your spokes, you'll make your bike sound like a motorcycle.

So, jump in the saddle, put your pedals to the metal and take this tiny tome on the open road from the comfort of your own home. Enjoy the ride!

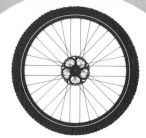

CHAPTER
ONE

Sweet Elevation

There's nothing like getting on your bike to solve all of the world's problems. And, remember, the higher you climb, the more fun it is on the way down. Take your brain on a ride and soak up the sweat of cyclists who have been to hell and back... their words are eternal.

"

When your legs
scream stop and
your lungs are
bursting, that's when
it starts. That's the
hurt locker. Winners
love it in there.

"

Chris McCormack

It was in 1888 that Scotsman John Dunlop invented the first practical pneumatic* tyre.

Source: CyclingUphill.com

*The puncture repair kit was invented in 1921.

Cyclophobia / bicyclophobia

The fear of riding a bicycle, commonly triggered after falling off a bike or crashing a bike.

Bonk

The moment that a cyclist experiences "hitting the wall", having used up all their energy due to glycogen depletion (glycogen is the fuel that's stored in your muscles).

"

To me, it doesn't matter
whether it's raining
or the sun is shining
or whatever: as long
as I'm riding a bike I
know I'm the luckiest
guy in the world.

"

Mark Cavendish

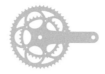

> ❝ When my legs hurt, I say: 'Shut up legs! Do what I tell you to do!' ❞

Jens Voigt

Playlist: Classics

1. *Riding on My Bike* – Madness
2. *The Bike Song* – Mark Ronson
3. *Bicycle* – John Cale
4. *Bicycle Race* – Queen
5. *Broken Bicycles* – Tom Waits
6. *Bicycle Song* – Red Hot Chili Peppers
7. *Bike* – Pink Floyd
8. *Silver Machine* – Hawkwind
9. *Nine Million Bicycles* – Katie Melua
10. *Riding on My Bike* – Sia

Englishman John Kemp Starley, in 1885, established the basic template for the modern bicycle. It was the first bicycle to feature two equal-sized wheels connected to a chain drive.

As long as I breathe, I attack.

Bernard Hinault

Cadence

A cyclist's pedalling rate, or the number of revolutions per minute (RPM).

"

Cyclists live with pain. If you can't handle it, you will win nothing.

"

Eddy Merckx

In 1817, Karl von Drais, the German baron widely acknowledged as the father of the bicycle, invented the first steerable, two-wheeled contraption. It had no chain, brakes or pedals.

"

It is the unknown around the corner that turns my wheels.

"

Heinz Stücke

"

Nothing
compares to the
simple pleasure
of riding a bike.

"

John F. Kennedy

"

Life is like riding a bicycle. To keep your balance, you must keep moving.

"

Albert Einstein

There are more than one billion bicycles currently in use around the world.

Source: WorldCycleTours.com

Drafting

The strategy of cycling behind another rider so they block the wind for you. Cyclists like to take advantage of this because it requires about 30 per cent less energy. Drafting behind a vehicle is called motorpacing.

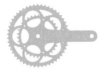

Give a man a fish and feed him for a day. Teach a man to fish and feed him for a lifetime. Teach a man to cycle and he will realize fishing is stupid and boring.

Desmond Tutu

The direct ancestor
of the modern bicycle
was the velocipede,
an iron and wood
construction invented
in the 1860s by the
Michaux family
of Paris. Its lack of
suspension earned
it the nickname
"boneshaker".

In the UK, two thirds of adults feel that it is too dangerous to cycle on the roads.

Source: Gov.UK

A human cycling on a bike can travel three times faster than they could walk for the same amount of energy.

(No other living thing on the planet can expend so little energy for so much self-powered travel.)

Source: ActionAid

66

It doesn't matter if you're sprinting for an Olympic gold medal, a town sign, a trailhead or the rest stop with the homemade brownies. If you never confront pain, you're missing the essence of the sport.

99

Scott Martin

A 2014 psychological study by the British Heart Foundation found that cyclists are 13 per cent more intelligent and cooler – and 10 per cent more charitable – than non-cyclists.

Source: *The Independent*

The health benefits of cycling outweigh the safety risks by a factor of 20 to one.

Source: Gov.UK

"

When the spirits are low, when the day appears dark, when work becomes monotonous, when hope hardly seems worth having, just mount a bicycle and go out for a spin down the road, without thought on anything but the ride you are taking.

Sir Arthur Conan Doyle

Globally, bike manufacturers produce approximately 100 million new bikes every year.

Source: WorldCycleTours.com

The newspaper that founded the Tour de France in 1903, *L'Auto*, was printed on yellow paper – hence the reason a yellow jersey is awarded to the race's leader. The same is true for Italy's tour, Giro d'Italia; the leader's jersey is pink, because sponsor *La Gazzetta dello Sport* was printed on pink paper.

Source: Bicycling.com

66

The bicycle is just as good company as most husbands and, when it gets old and shabby, a woman can dispose of it and get a new one without shocking the entire community.

99

Ann Strong

66

You can say that
climbers suffer the
same as the other
riders, but they suffer
in a different way.
You feel the pain,
but you're glad to
be there.

Richard Virenque

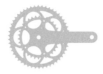

"

Riding a bike is everything to a cyclist. The friendship and camaraderie you have with other cyclists... to a cyclist, it was the be-all and end-all of your life.

Tommy Godwin

It is estimated that more than 1.5 billion people watch the Tour de France on TV during the three weeks of broadcast coverage, across 190 countries, making it the third most-viewed sport event in the world.

Source: BBC

> The best rides are the ones where you bite off much more than you can chew, and live through it.

Doug Bradbury

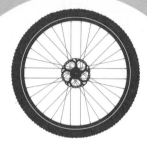

CHAPTER
TWO

Wheels on Fire

Wheels have fascinated the human mind ever since they were invented. And, as ever, two is better than one. A bicycle is more than just a metal machine made of gears, cables and wheels. It's a symbol of revolution...

"

Bicycling is a big part of the future. It has to be. There's something wrong with a society that drives a car to work out in a gym.

"

Bill Nye

The bicycle is a curious vehicle. Its passenger is its engine.

John Howard

"

Truly, the
bicycle is the
most influential
piece of product
design ever.

"

Hugh Pearman

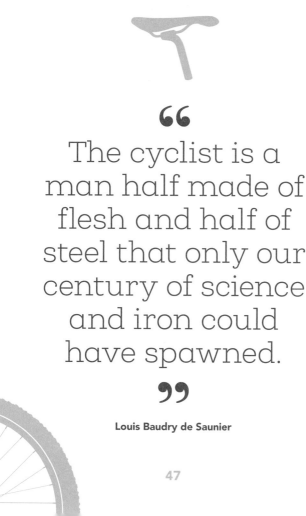

"

The cyclist is a man half made of flesh and half of steel that only our century of science and iron could have spawned.

"

Louis Baudry de Saunier

66

Cyclists see considerably more of this beautiful world than any other class of citizens. A good bicycle, well applied, will cure most ills this flesh is heir to.

99

K.K. Doty

In the Tour's earliest races, the bikes that Tour de France cyclists used going up the mountains weighed 40 pounds (18kg) each. Today, bikes weigh in at 15 pounds (6.8kg), but never any less than that.

Source: Bicycling.com

"

You always know
when you're going to
arrive. If you go by car,
you don't. Apart from
anything else, I prefer
cycling. It puts you in
a good mood, I find.

"

Alan Bennett

The derailleur system was introduced in the Tour de France for the first time in 1937, though it was in 1949 when the first refined cable-operated rear derailleur was introduced. Cyclists now no longer needed to stop halfway up a mountain to change gear.

Source: BikeRadar.com

"

The bicycle is the most civilized conveyance known to man. Other forms of transport grow daily more nightmarish. Only the bicycle remains pure in heart.

"

Iris Murdoch

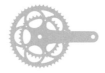

66

Learn to ride a bicycle. You will not regret it if you live.

99

Mark Twain

"

When I was a kid
I used to pray every
night for a new
bicycle. Then I realized
that the Lord doesn't
work that way so I
stole one and asked
Him to forgive me.

Emo Philips

66

Ride as much or
as little, as long
or as short as
you feel. But ride.

99

Eddy Merckx

66

Life is like a ten-speed bicycle. Most of us have gears we never use.

99

Charles M. Schulz

66
Bicycles are almost as good as guitars for meeting girls. 99

Bob Weir

66

Crashing is part of cycling as crying is part of love.

99

Johan Museeuw

66
You are one ride
away from a
good mood.
99

Sarah Bentley

During the Tour de France, the 20 or so competing international teams of nine riders cycle more than 2,200 miles (3,500km), on various routes that alternate between clockwise and counterclockwise circuits of France.

Source: BikeRadar.com

Playlist: Blood, Sweat and Gears

1. *Tour de France* - Kraftwerk
2. *Freewheel Burning* - Judas Priest
3. *Hold On* – Santana
4. *Chains* - Tina Arena
5. *Gears of War* – Megadeth
6. *Back in the Saddle* - Aerosmith
7. *Open Road* - Bryan Adams
8. *Yellow* - Coldplay
9. *Road Rage* - Catatonia
10. *Take Me Home, Country Roads* - John Denver

The average Tour de France rider burns an average of 6,000 calories per day! Over the course of the 21-day race that's approximately 126,000 calories.

Source: *Cycling Weekly*

It never gets easier, you just get faster.

Greg LeMond

"

One of the most important days of my life was when I learned to ride a bicycle.

"

Michael Palin

Over the course of the roughly 2,200-mile (3,500km) Tour de France, a cyclist will sweat about 3 pints (1.5 litres) per hour, totalling 34 gallons (130 litres) for the entire race. That's a lot of sweat, enough to flush a toilet over 20 times at 1.6 gallons (6 litres) per flush.

Source: BikeRadar.com

66

If you brake, you don't win.

99

Mario Cipollini

66

Whenever I see an adult on a bicycle, I do not despair for the human race.

99

H.G. Wells

66

If constellations had been named in the 20th century, I suppose we would see bicycles.

Carl Sagan

Biking at a speed of 12–14 miles (20–22km) per hour will cause a 155-pound (70kg) person to burn 298 calories in 30 minutes – roughly the same calories in a McDonald's cheeseburger (though they can be eaten in less than a minute!).

Source: Harvard University

Endo

When a rider flips head over heels over the handlebars, end over end – endo.

The interaction of the body, mind, muscles, terrain, gravity, air and bicycle are so complex that they defy exact mathematical solutions. The feel and handling of a bike borders on art.

Chester Kyle

> **"**
>
> # Those who wish to control their own lives and move beyond existence as mere clients and consumers – those people ride a bike.
>
> **"**

Wolfgang Sachs

66

A bicycle ride around the world begins with a single pedal stroke.

99

Scott Stoll

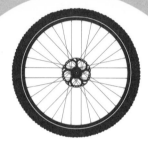

CHAPTER
THREE

Revolution in the Head

It's impossible to feel sad on a bike, so they say. The rush of wind, the feeling of flying, the elevated pulse of a heartbeat – cycling is a drug, as addictive as love. But like love, sometimes it can be heartbreaking...

"

You can't get good by staying home. If you want to get fast, you have to go where the fast guys are.

"

Steve Larsen

**

The bicycle is
the most efficient
machine ever created.
Converting calories
into gas, a bicycle
gets the equivalent
of 3,000 miles
per gallon.

"

Bill Strickland

66

Riding bicycles will not only benefit the individual doing it, but the world at large.

99

Udo E. Simonis

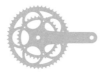

"

Commuting by bicycle is an absolutely essential part of my day. It's mind-clearing, invigorating. I get to go out and pedal through the countryside in the early morning hours, and see life come back and rejuvenate every day as the sun is coming out.

"

James L. Jones

More than 12 million spectators gather to line the routes of the Tour de France, making it the largest spectator sporting event in the world.

Source: *The Guardian*

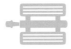

"

Meet the future; the future mode of transportation for this weary Western world. Now I'm not gonna make a lot of extravagant claims for this little machine. Sure, it'll change your whole life for the better, but that's all.

"

Henry Jones, as the bicycle salesman in *Butch Cassidy and the Sundance Kid* (1969)

Ned Flanders:
"You were bicycling two abreast?"

Homer Simpson:
"I wish. We were bicycling to a lake."

The Simpsons, "Dangerous Curves", Season 20, Episode 5, written by Billy Kimball and Ian Maxtone-Graham

The first winner of the Tour de France in 1903 was a chimney sweeper – Maurice Garin. "I had trouble on the road," Garin said after the race. "I was hungry, I was thirsty, I was sleepy, I suffered. I cried between Lyon and Marseille."

Source: Cyclist.co.uk

"

An engineer designing
from scratch could
hardly concoct a
better device than
a bicycle to unclog
modern roads –
cheap, non-polluting,
small and silent...

"

Rick Smith

66

Cyclists are more civic-minded than anyone else travelling in any other manner, bar by foot. If they do run into someone, they at least (like the bee) do their victim the favour of hurting themselves in the process.

99

Zoe Williams

The overall average speed of recent Tour de France riders is 25 miles (40km) per hour – though obviously speeds differ for uphill, downhill, time trials, flatland. This is the same speed as a charging elephant.

Source: WorldCycleTours.com

"

Few articles ever
used by man have
created so great
a revolution in
social conditions
as the bicycle.

"

US Census Bureau Report, 1900

"

Bicycling... is the nearest approximation I know to the flight of birds.

"

Louis J. Halle

> Man on a bicycle can go three or four times faster than the pedestrian, but uses five times less energy in the process. Equipped with this tool, man outstrips the efficiency of not only all machines but all other animals as well.

Ivan Illich

"

There may be a better land where bicycle saddles are made of rainbow, stuffed with cloud; in this world the simplest thing is to get used to something hard.

Jerome K. Jerome

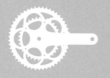

A bicycle is an industrial revolution in an individual's life.

F. K. Day

"

When man invented
the bicycle, he
reached the peak
of his attainments.
Progress should have
stopped when man
invented the bicycle.

"

Elizabeth West

66

A bicycle does get you there and more. And there is always the thin edge of danger to keep you alert and comfortably apprehensive. And getting there is all the fun.

99

Bill Emerson

There are three annual races that define the Grand Tour: the Tour de France (France), the Giro d'Italia (Italy) and the Vuelta a España (Spain). They are all three weeks long and involve a mix of individual and team time trials, mountain climbs and sprints that total more than 2,000 miles (3,218km).

66

Newspapers are unable, seemingly, to discriminate between a bicycle accident and the collapse of civilization.

George Bernard Shaw

"

A bicycle is an unparalleled merger of a toy, a utilitarian vehicle and sporting equipment.

,,

Bill Strickland

> **A woman needs a man like a fish needs a bicycle.**

Irina Dunn

66

A person pedalling a bike uses energy more efficiently than an eagle. And a triangle-framed bicycle can easily carry ten times its own weight – a capacity no automobile, airplane or bridge can match.

99

Bill Strickland

"

After a long day on my bicycle, I feel refreshed, cleansed, purified. I feel that I have established contact with my environment and that I am at peace. On days like that, I am permeated with a profound gratitude for my bicycle...

"

Paul de Vivie

66

In politics, one can learn some things from cycling, such as how to have character and courage. Sometimes in politics there isn't enough of those things.

99

Guy Verhofstadt

Marriage is a wonderful invention: then again, so is a bicycle repair kit.

Billy Connolly

A rider is about six times heavier than their bike.

(A car is 20 times heavier than you.)

Source: BikeRadar.com

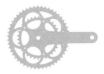

"

Cycling for everyone
has more defeat than
victory, more pain
than wellness, more
effort than glory, but
all of that combined
makes cycling so
fascinating.

Rubens Bertogliati

"

Bicycles may change, but cycling is timeless.

"

Zapata Espinoza

> **"**
>
> You never have the wind with you – either it is against you or you're having a good day.
>
> **"**

Daniel Behrman

“

There is nothing,
absolutely
nothing, quite so
worthwhile as
simply messing
about on bicycles.

”

Tom Kunich

"
Like dogs,
bicycles are social
catalysts that
attract a superior
category of people.
"

Chip Brown

Granny Gear

The lowest gear ratio possible on your bike – the smallest chainring in the front and the largest chainring in the back. Essential for elevation climbs, useless on flats.

"

Cycle tracks
will abound
in Utopia.

"

H.G. Wells

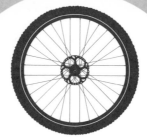

CHAPTER
FOUR

Head over Heels

Riding a bike is not just like riding a bike – no matter what your parents say. Cycling requires focus, attention and dedication, no matter whether you're popping to the shops, climbing a mountain or flat-out on a time trial. These cyclists and pro-riders know the pain. Do you?

66

Bicycles have no walls.

99

Paul Cornish

The first commercially sold bicycle – known as a "boneshaker" – weighed 176 pounds (80kg) when it first appeared on sale in Paris in 1868.

Source: WorldCycleTours.com

"

Pain is still the friend that always tells me the truth.

"

Chris Froome

Training is like fighting with a gorilla. You don't stop when you're tired. You stop when the gorilla is tired.

Greg Henderson

"

Cycling isn't a game, it's a sport. Tough, hard and unpitying, and it requires great sacrifices. One plays football, or tennis, or hockey. One doesn't play at cycling.

"

Jean de Gribaldy

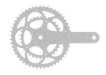

66

Beyond pain there is a whole universe of more pain.

99

Jens Voigt

66

I have always struggled to achieve excellence. One thing that cycling has taught me is that if you can achieve something without a struggle it's not going to be satisfying.

Greg LeMond

The Netherlands
is the so-called
bicycle capital of
the world, with
upwards of 22.5
million bicycles for
a population of
17 million.

Source: BicycleDutch.wordpress.com

"

Cycling throws up plenty of obstacles, unknown territory, high-speed split-second considerations. Where to next? What's around the next corner? Who cares? You're flyin'!

"

Cadel Evans

"

Good morale in cycling comes from good legs.

"

Sean Yates

"

You either love
spinning the pedals
and watching scenery
whiz by, or you don't.
And if you love it, not
much can sour you
on the idea of riding
your bike.

"

Keith Mills

Your bike is discovery;
your bike is freedom.
It doesn't matter
where you are, when
you're on the saddle,
you're taken away.

Doug Donaldson

"

...if you have ever, just once, sat on a bicycle with a singing heart and felt like an ordinary human touching the gods, then we share something fundamental. We know it's all about the bike.

"

Robert Penn

Around 20 million bicycles are sold in the United States annually.

(Mountain bikes were the most popular category, as of 2019.)

Source: Statista.com

"

Ride a bike.
Ride a bike.
Ride a bike.

"

Fausto Coppi

A mountain bike is like your buddy. A road bike is your lover.

Sean Coffey

> "
>
> # If you do something right the first time, then it's not hard enough.
>
> "

Danny MacAskill

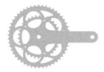

66

My two favourite things in life are libraries and bicycles. They both move people forward without wasting anything.

Peter Golkin

"

Cycling has encountered more enemies than any other form of exercise.

"

Louis Baudry de Saunier

"

I promise I will never be in a bicycle race. That I can tell you.

"

Donald Trump

❝

What's with these recumbent bicycles? Listen, buddy, if you wanna take a nap, lie down. If you wanna ride a bike, buy a fucking bicycle.

❞

George Carlin

66

I thought of
that while riding
my bicycle.

99

Albert Einstein (on the Theory of Relativity)

"

When I go biking I am mentally far, far away from civilization. The world is breaking someone else's heart.

"

Diane Ackerman

Bicycles save over 238 million gallons (1,082 litres) of fuel every year.

Source: WorldCycleTours.com

"

I love the bicycle. I always have. I can think of no sincere, decent human being, male or female, young or old, saintly or sinful, who can resist the bicycle.

"

William Saroyan

The bicycle has a soul. If you succeed to love it, it will give you emotions that you will never forget.

Mario Cipollini

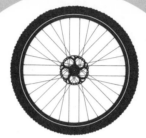

CHAPTER
FIVE

Grand Tour

From competitive cycling to tour riding, and mountain biking to city commuting, every rider yearns for the open road to take them home. Life is about the journey, not the destination, after all. What's your Grand Tour?

"

The journey of life is like a man riding a bicycle. We know he got on the bicycle and started to move. We know that at some point he will stop and get off. We know that if he stops moving and does not get off, he will fall off.

"

William Golding

> My legs and a silly something in me cry out for knocking the milestones down one by one and stopping at nothing. For years I have been telling myself that it's not the mile in the life that counts, but the life in the miles. But still this silly restlessness hurries me on.

Harold Elvin

"

Maybe, deep down, cyclists know that hills, and the temporary pain and struggle they involve, are a fantastic metaphor for life. It's shit when you're struggling. But the pain will end. It always does. There's always a summit. You've just got to keep going.

Mike Carter

Anyone who rides a bike is a friend of mine.

Gary Fisher

"

Gliding down the bike path on a Saturday morning, you whip by somebody pedalling in the opposite direction and give each other a nod. For a moment it's like 'Hey, we're both doing the same thing. Let's be friends for a second.'

"

Neil Pasricha

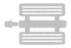

"

Striker, listen, and you listen close: flying a plane is no different than riding a bicycle, just a lot harder to put baseball cards in the spokes.

"

Robert Stack as Captain Rex Kramer,
Airplane! **(1980)**

"

Sex is like riding a bicycle. The first nine times you fall off, but the tenth time you can go on for miles.

"

Sean Patrick Flanery as Tom Bartlett,
Simply Irresistible (1999)

"

He rode his bicycle into a tree, C.J., what do you want me... The President, while riding his bicycle on his vacation in Jackson Hole, came to a sudden arboreal stop.

"

John Spencer as Leo McGarry,
The West Wing, "Pilot" (1999)

66

The future's all yours, you lousy bicycles.

99

Paul Newman as Butch Cassidy, *Butch Cassidy and the Sundance Kid* **(1969)**

66

The truth hurts, doesn't it? Oh sure, maybe not as much as jumping on a bicycle with the seat missing, but it hurts.

99

Leslie Nielsen as Frank Drebin, *The Naked Gun* (1988)

On average, cyclists live two years longer than non-cyclists. They also take 15 per cent fewer days off work through illness.

Source: European Cyclists' Federation

66

I know the
freedom that
cycling gives you
in terms of being
able to just jump
on and go.

99

Bradley Wiggins

"

Cycling is good for people in all ways: their health, their wellbeing, and it does no damage to the environment. It can, however, be dangerous, and this has to be addressed.

"

Jeremy Corbyn

In cycling, you just race. When you get to the finish, you see the result.

Pauline Ferrand-Prévot

"

I need to be on a bike, mentally as much as physically.

"

Mark Cavendish

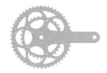

Bicycles are the most efficient vehicles on the planet, 50 times more efficient than cars, and twice as efficient as walking.

Godo Stoyke

An adult who cycles regularly will typically have a level of fitness equivalent to being ten years younger.

Source: European Cyclists' Federation

> **"**
> First week
> you feel good,
> the second
> week you lose
> strength. Third
> week, f*cked.
> **"**

Per Pedersen (about the Tour de France)

66

The problem with being a Tour de France winner is you always have the feeling of disappointment if you don't win it again. That's the curse of the Tour de France.

Greg LeMond

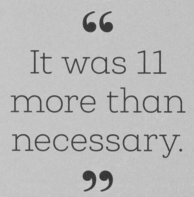

66

It was 11
more than
necessary.

99

**Jacques Anquetil (after winning a Tour de France
race by 12 seconds)**

"

It's the stuff of dreams. As a child, being a fan of the sport, I never imagined that one day I'd be in this position. Kids from Kilburn don't become favourite for the Tour de France. You're supposed to become a postman or a milkman or work in Ladbrokes.

Bradley Wiggins

I'm still that eight-year-old kid who rode up the Stelvio. I'm still that kid in my legs, in my head and in my heart.

Ivan Basso

“

To race a bike, you need to be a poor man.

”

Biagio Cavanna

No hour of life is lost that is spent in the saddle.

Winston Churchill

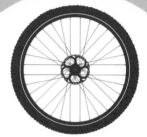

CHAPTER
SIX

Life Cycle

Pick yourself up. Put the book down. And go for a ride. We won't mind. Cycling is life! And these riders and bike lovers have seen the light...

"

There simply is nothing else
like the Tour de France. And, as
a test of physical and mental
endurance, it has no equal. Other
sports may be as intense, as
pressurized, as hard for short
periods, but the Tour goes on day
after day after day. It's the only
race in the world where you have
to get a haircut halfway through.

Chris Boardman

Variable gears are only for people over 45. Isn't it better to triumph by the strength of your muscles rather than by the artifice of a derailleur? We are getting soft. Give me a fixed gear.

Henri Desgrange (creator of the Tour de France, 1903)

Tour de France Legends

1. Eddy Merckx - Belgium
Five times winner: 1969, 1970, 1971, 1972 and 1974

2. Miguel Induráin - Spain
Five times winner: 1991, 1992, 1993, 1994 and 1995

3. Jacques Anquetil - France
Five times winner: 1957, 1961, 1962, 1963 and 1964

4. Lance Armstrong - USA
Seven times winner: 1999, 2000, 2001, 2002, 2003, 2004 and 2005

(All wins were stripped due to illegal doping.)

5. Bernard Hinault - France
Five times winner: 1978, 1979, 1981, 1982 and 1985

6. Greg LeMond - USA
Three times winner: 1986, 1989 and 1990

7. Chris Froome - UK
Two times winner: 2013 and 2015

8. Alberto Contador - Spain
Three times winner: 2007, 2009 and 2010

9. Philippe Thys - Belgium
Three times winner: 1913, 1914 and 1920

10. Fausto Coppi - Italy
Two times winner: 1949 and 1952

Source: *Cycling Weekly*

"

Running would be much better if they invented a little seat to sit on... Oh wait.

"

Liz Hatch

> Bike riding is a beautiful thing. Peaceful and serene, flowing and artistic, freeing and blissful, pedalling a bike over hill and dale is ethereal. Tack a number on your back, though, and bike racing is a bizarrely unnatural sport hinging so much on luck.

Ted King

Drivetrain

The entire mechanical system – pedals, cranks, front and rear derailleurs, chainrings, cassette and chain – that converts pedalling into forward momentum. The drivetrain is your bike's engine.

"

Cycling is such a stupid sport. Next time you are in a car travelling at 40mph think about jumping out – naked. That's what it's like when we crash.

"

David Millar

"

The bicycle, the bicycle surely, should always be the vehicle of novelists and poets.

"

Christopher Morley

My biggest fear is not crashing on a bike... It's sitting in a chair at 90 and saying, 'I wish I had done more'.

Graeme Obree

"

Every downhill, every road, every flat piece of road, every finish line we're doing 60km an hour; it's a dangerous sport. We accept that. It's just the way it is.

"

Dan Martin

"

I know I'm pushing the boundaries. I know that one of these days I'm going to hit the dust and I'm going to be fucking history, but sod it.

"

Sean Yates

66

You can't ride the Tour de France on mineral water.

99

Jacques Anquetil

66

Everybody wants to know what I'm on. What am I on? I'm on my bike busting my ass six hours a day. What are you on?

Lance Armstrong

Peloton

The largest
pack of riders
in a road race.
A pack of riders
stick together to
allow cyclists to
take advantage
of drafting.

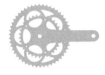

To prepare for a race there is nothing better than a good pheasant, some champagne and a woman.

Jacques Anquetil

66

Every race is a war. Every race is a fight. If you don't go into every event with that belief, you will never achieve your goals.

99

Fabian Cancellara

I race to win, not to please people.

Bernard Hinault

"

Cycling is suffering.

"

Fausto Coppi

> **"**
> # If it hurts me, it must hurt the other ones twice as much.
> **"**

Jens Voigt

66

Cycling is quite a pure sport: it is mainly about suffering, whether you are climbing the Tourmalet, racing up Mont Ventoux, or trying to survive in Paris-Roubaix.

Bradley Wiggins

"

The best that can be said of the hill climb is, as philosopher Thomas Hobbes wrote of human life, that it is 'nasty, brutish and short'.

"

Matt Seaton

"

You don't suffer, kill yourself and take the risks I take just for money. I love bike racing.

"

Greg LeMond

LSD

Long steady/
slow distance.
LSD refers to a
lengthy training
ride at a constant
aerobic pace.

66

I don't mind what people say about my style. If it's the quickest way to get from A to B, that's how we're going to do it.

99

Chris Froome

> **"**
> Real heroes are
> others, those who have
> suffered in their soul,
> in their heart, in their
> spirit, in their mind, for
> their loved ones. Those
> are the real heroes. I'm
> just a cyclist.
> **"**

Gino Bartali

66

I do want to be a
spokesman for clean
cycling – I believe
somebody has to
stand up for the
current generation.
I'm happy to do that.

99

Chris Froome